DELIVER!

*A concise guide to helping the
woman you love through labor*

by
Julie Dubrouillet & Simon Firth

Deliver! Books

Copyright 2012 Julie Dubrouillet and Simon Firth
Version 1.41, Feb. 2012
Published by Deliver Books, Palo Alto, CA.
Visit: www.deliverbook.com

ISBN 10: 0985256419
ISBN 13: 978-0-9852564-1-8

Illustrations by Sara Burgess
(www.whitepaperspress.com)

Legal notice
*This book is for informational and educational use only. Any
advice or recommendations herein do not constitute medical
advice, practice, diagnosis or treatment, nor is it intended to
replace the necessity of a consultation with your physician or
other medical practitioner.*

Praise for *Deliver! A concise guide to helping the woman you love through labor:*

"Deliver! is very good. It's concise and medically accurate. Most importantly, it's all about how partners/spouses and medical staff can best support expectant moms - the approach that we should universally adopt as providers for women in labor."

Winona M. Tan, M.D. Palo Alto Medical Foundation, Obstetrics and Gynecology, Board Certified

Table of contents

INTRODUCTION
About the Book and its Authors

Why we wrote this book

Modern men are almost universally expected to attend the birth of their children. But too often they have no idea what to do during labor. Without a clear sense of their role, men can see someone they love in great distress and feel powerless to help. Meanwhile laboring women, unless they feel fully supported by everyone around them, risk slowing or even stalling their progress, which in turn risks increased – and otherwise unneeded – medical intervention. The consequences of a poorly supported birth can be long-lasting, even to the point of severely straining the relationship that brought the baby into the world.

But men and women can do the just opposite, of course. Together, they can help make a birth a wonderfully positive event that builds on – and strengthens – the love and trust that is at the heart of their relationship.

And yet while birth books for women abound, the resources available to men to explain exactly what they can do to help are few and unsatisfactory. Expectant mothers commonly complain to us that their partners don't read the books they give them – because what's available is too long, too sophomoric or simply not written with men in mind.

Finally, help is at hand. *Deliver! Helping the woman you love through labor* is a concise, straight-talking field guide to birth written expressly for men. We take fathers-to-be through the various stages of labor and birth, clearly explaining what a woman is experiencing and – most importantly – suggesting the many ways in which their partners can help.

Okay, it's not just for men

We've addressed this book to men because in the vast majority of cases it is a man who will be accompanying the laboring mom in the delivery room. And most often that man is also the father of the baby.

But sisters can make wonderful birth partners, as can girlfriends (and guy friends) and even moms and grandmoms, dads and granddads.

If you're a female birth partner and reading this book, sorry for all the 'he's and 'him's – we hope you can get some good ideas from this, too. Certainly, there's nothing we suggest here that requires a Y chromosome to do it.

How you want to give birth is your choice

Some birth books have very strong ideas about where exactly you should give birth. This one doesn't. We don't care if you want to give birth at home, in a hot tub, hanging from a trapeze or in the more typical setting of the Labor and Delivery ward at your local hospital. As far as we're concerned, they can all be a good choice (well, except maybe the trapeze…).

What we're about is supporting the laboring mom in the choices she has made and in the circumstances in which she finds herself as she gives birth to her child – which, after all, don't always turn out to be the same thing.

This book is meant to be a quick read.

We know people are busy. We know that birth partners often don't have the time or the inclination to pick up long, detailed books about childbirth – or attend multi-week birthing classes.

And we know that there are many excellent books that cover every eventuality and medical obscurity that you could possibly encounter. We point you to some of our favorites at our website: www.deliverbook.com.

What we're offering here, though, are the basics – the things that are most likely to be of most use to most people.
This is a living document, however. If there's stuff you really wanted us to cover and that you couldn't find in here, let us know. You can reach us at deliverbook@yahoo.com. We'll try to add it in the next edition.

Who we are

Julie is a certified labor support doula, childbirth and lactation educator and prenatal yoga instructor, as well as a trainer of childbirth educators. She is also the pre-natal Health Education Specialist at the Palo Alto Medical Foundation in Palo Alto, California. A mother of two children, she's taught thousands of couples how best to approach childbirth and directly supported hundreds of couples through the births of their children.

Simon is a writer specializing in stories about parenting and technology. He's written for Salon, Wondertime, Food and Wine and the Christian Science Monitor among other publications and is a regular technology analyst for the London Evening Standard. He attended the births of his two children, where he lovingly supported his wife thanks to the tips he learned in a class taught by Julie! Julie was also the doula attending his children's births.

Send us feedback

Again, this is a living document. We want it to keep getting better and better. So let us know what you think could make it even more helpful. Write to us at deliverbook@yahoo.com and tell us what else you'd like us to cover or how else we could be a help.

WHY LABOR SUPPORT

CHAPTER ONE

Support, whatever your choice

You are going to have a baby. Congratulations!

You're now over that first rush of excitement, perhaps. You're far enough along to tell your friends and family. And you're realizing that it really isn't that long before this baby is going to be born.

That means you need to make some decisions about how you'd like it to happen.

In some cases it's already a foregone conclusion: there's a medical reason to schedule a C-section right now; or everything looks normal and you're 100% planning for a home birth.

Most people, though, are somewhere in the middle. In this book, we're not going to weigh in on home-births versus hospital births or epidurals versus *au naturale*. That's all up to you. Our concern is that the mom-to-be will be supported – however she and her partner have chosen to make that happen.

So, why labor support?

We sometimes hear expectant moms say something like, "the labor isn't so important to me, I'm just interested in having a healthy baby." Fair enough, to a degree. What does really matter in the end is for both baby and mom to emerge from the process healthy and ready to fall in love with each other.

But just because labor seems like a means to an end doesn't mean it isn't important – or that the choices couples make about it won't have an impact on how ready the mom, baby and even the father will be for the daunting next stage of helping their baby grow up in the world.

Better instead to think of labor as an event in its own right. It's like the difference between a wedding and a marriage. A wedding is really just what you need to go through to be married. But no-one would argue that weddings aren't important events on their own.

Similarly, labor is the passage to becoming a parent and a traumatic birth – like a traumatic wedding – is worth trying to avoid.

Even if this is your first birth, you likely already know this. Maybe you have friends or relatives who came out of childbirth with a healthy baby but deeply upset by the process in some way. Perhaps the birth was longer or more painful than they expected, perhaps they had an unplanned C-section, or perhaps they were anxious and fearful and they couldn't find the support they needed from their partner or hospital staff.

Often when women try to talk about these feelings, family and friends are unsympathetic. "But you have a healthy baby," they suggest, "why be upset?" And women will often feel guilty or ungrateful for feeling that way. Obviously, though, neither the initial experience nor those unsympathetic responses and the upset they provoke are at all helpful.

Indeed, research shows that women who feel better about their labor experience:
- Feel a closer bond with their baby AND their partner
- Have less postpartum depression
- Are more likely to have successful breastfeeding experiences

Making labor and birth a positive experience

So what makes someone feel better about their birth experience?

In years of talking to women about labor and birth, we've found that usually it's not the outcome that dictates their feelings about either, but the experience itself. It's about what happened to their plans for medication as their labor progressed, for example, and whether they felt listened to. It's about how their hopes for a vaginal delivery, or avoiding an episiotomy, or having a home birth, were respected and supported, even when medical circumstances forced those plans to be put aside.

The bottom line: Women who feel they were taken care of, respected and listened to will typically look back at labor as a positive experience. And that in turn can make a huge difference to those first few key weeks and months postpartum.

Labor support, in other words, is of enormous value.

Doulas – the professional birth partner

It's for this reason that many couples choose to have a doula with them at their birth. Doulas are, in essence, professional labor supporters. They act as experienced advocates for the laboring mother in the face of what can often be a confusing, impersonal, medicalized birthing process that focuses almost exclusively on physical health in ways that can unnecessarily, and avoidably, make for a traumatic birth experience for the mom.

Many birth partners – even if they plan to be present for their partner at the birth – want to have a doula present as well. It's their first child, perhaps. Or he's anxious, or feels uncomfortable knowing he'll be the sole support during a process that can last many hours. So they hire a doula.

A good doula will welcome a partner's presence and help him support the woman he loves – even as the doula is being a support as well. She'll suggest – and employ herself – many of the techniques and tips in this book.

Doulas are wonderful and we've both hired doulas ourselves and would again. They're welcomed by good doctors, too, who've read the numerous studies that show the positive benefits that doulas bring to childbirth.

But not everyone feels comfortable having a hired labor supporter present at the time of birth – or has the resources to do so.

You the labor partner – you can deliver!

This book is for those couples as well as for couples who do engage a doula. Whatever the combination of professionals helping out (doulas, midwives, doctors and nurses), we want to help birth partners be more supportive and better advocates for the women they love as they undergo the extraordinary experience of labor and childbirth.

As we said in the introduction, no woman and no birth is the same. It would take a shelf-full of books to cover all the possible situations that births can provoke. Those books, and many more, already exist.

It is possible, though, to offer set of clear, succinct instructions and advice that all couples should know and think about going into childbirth - and that we're confident will be very helpful. That's what we're offering here.

THE LAST FEW MONTHS
CHAPTER TWO

Here's where we start: You're past the first trimester. You're both moving from focusing on how to keep your baby healthy in utero to wondering how exactly you'll bring this growing little person into the world.

It's decision time

You're probably reading this having already made some fundamental choices about how you would like your baby to be born - a hospital versus a home birth, medication versus toughing-it-out, or midwife-led deliveries versus an OB-led birth. If you haven't decided, now really is the time to be thinking about which of these choices you're going to make. It's worth remembering, though, that as you progress through the pregnancy, either of you may realize that you aren't comfortable with the path you are on, or with the people you have chosen to help. If that happens, it's almost never too late to make the changes you need to make you feel safe and comfortable.

If you do still need to make some of your fundamental birthing decisions, or want to confirm that they're the right ones for you, read through the next three chapters. They look at some of options you have on issues like pain medication, that you might want to explore ahead of time. Overall, this is a good time to discuss how you'd like things to go with whomever you're considering adding to your birthing team (the next chapter looks at writing birth plans, for example, as well as birth teams).

The bottom line: it's always her call

Here's a message that we'll be coming back to again and again, because it's both true and also the most important thing to remember in being a great birth supporter: in the end, the one with the baby inside gets to make the call.

Where to give birth, how to give birth, with whom to give birth – in the end, they're all up to her.

She'll want to know what you think. She'll really appreciate talking with you, hearing about the research you've been able to do, knowing that you are there to listen to her worries and concerns. But she's the one who'll be most directly affected here, so after all's said and done, she gets to decide.

And once her decision is made, your job is to support her in that choice, even if you would do things differently yourself. That's not because this isn't about you – if you're the father of the child, or even if you just care very much for her, of course you're affected too.

It's because feeling supported will make the birth a much more positive experience for her – and that, as we said in the last chapter, can make a huge difference to the outcome of the birth. It can impact the long term health of the mother and child, and the quality of your relationship with them both once there's a new baby to love and raise.

Lecture over

So, you've decided where you'd like to give birth and established how you are going to be making decisions together. Her due date is likely still a few months away, but there are several things you can be doing right now to improve your chances of a smooth labor.

Take a class

This is the time to think about what else, besides reading this book, you can be doing by way of pre-birth homework.

Traditionally, what most expecting couples have done is take a class.

For decades now, the childbirth class has been a rite of passage for pregnant couples. We're all familiar with the sitcom favorite of room full of pregnant couples sitting around on pillows huffing and puffing. But, for all their comic potential – and the time they take to attend – these classes have plenty going for them.

The straight dope

Their most obvious value is informational. A series run by your local hospital, medical clinic or local birthing center will tell you pretty much everything you need to know about your options for where to give birth, when to go to the hospital or call the midwife, what to expect during the birth itself and the medical options you're likely to be presented with. A good class will also focus on our main subject here – how to be a great labor supporter. We see birth classes as complementary to, not in competition with, what we're offering here.

There are some less obvious benefits, too, especially for first-time parents:

1) The chance to come together as a couple
In our busy lives, it can sometimes be hard to find time to focus on each other and the upcoming event. Classes give you that time. With luck, they'll also open up conversations about both of your expectations, hopes and fears – conversations you really want to be having around now.

2) Finding community
Of course there is no guarantee that you'll make lifelong friends in childbirth class, but we see it happen all the time. Classes put you in a group of relative neighbors who are in your exact same life space, all about to cross over from couple-hood to parenthood. Though you may be very different in many ways, being in this same place levels many differences. You're bound to like at least some of the parents you meet in the class, which makes them natural candidates to join you in a parent-and-baby group once your babies are born.

Other kinds of classes

Yoga: Physical preparation for a physical activity

A lot of modern childbirth prep is directed at a woman's mental state, even though labor and birth are, obviously, extremely physical. Practicing birth-specific yoga goes a long way to help redress that balance. Remember, you don't have to be a Yogini (or to have ever taken a yoga class for that matter), to start, and reap huge benefit from, prenatal yoga.

During pregnancy, yoga helps alleviate physical discomforts such as back and hip pain, and helps with insomnia and relaxation. As preparation for labor it teaches women to be present with and breathe through discomfort, as well as relaxing into sensations that may feel hard to manage. Women often report to us that their prenatal yoga class was the single most helpful thing they did to get through pregnancy and the birth process.

Breastfeeding class: The big suck

Another class that we highly recommend is breastfeeding. This is nature's own and best method for nourishing a human infant, but it's not wholly instinctive. It's a learned process that in the past was acquired by watching women in the community throughout our childhoods. These days, most women need to learn it some other way. With breastfeeding, the old adage 'forewarned is forearmed' really applies. The more a woman understands in advance about how it works, the more likely it is that her efforts will proceed smoothly.

If you skip the classes, do your own research

If you decide that classes really aren't for you, this is the time to get to the library, bookstore, or the internet and do research of your own. And to read this book, of course!

The 'Recommended' section of our website, www.deliverbook.com, links to some of the best books currently available on pregnancy, birth, birth support and parenting, as well as reputable websites covering similar topics.

Then tour the labor ward

It's also a good idea for you both to go and see where your baby will be born. Hospitals have particular rules and routines that you should know about. Even if you took a class that covered them, it's great to see where you'll be going before you turn up in mid-labor.

When you're there, don't be afraid to ask questions. Whatever's concerning you is likely to be worrying most of the other people there, too. They'll thank you for being the one to speak up!

If you are planning to give birth at home, you still need to make ready for the birth. Your doctor or midwife has no doubt already given you a list of the things you'll need – now's the time to go buy them.

Birth apps – worth a dollar

A variety of birth-related phone and tablet apps are now available to help you and your partner in all kinds of ways as you prepare for childbirth. They'll manage appointments, track weight, nutrition, medications and even help count the baby's kicks. Come the onset of labor, they can monitor contractions, and offer lists of what you need to take with you to the delivery room.

One of our favorite apps is the Pregnancy Companion created by Drs. Jan Rydfors and Aron Schuftan of the Bay Area Fertility and Pregnancy Specialists group. It does everything listed above, and more, for just 99c.

THE LAST FEW WEEKS
CHAPTER THREE

The baby's due date is now just a few weeks off. The little one will likely be kicking up a storm. Your partner will probably have already felt some stronger Braxton Hicks, or 'practice,' contractions (they start as early as six weeks into a pregnancy, but aren't usually felt until much later on).

What you want now is for the baby to begin positioning him- or herself for birth. Positioned right, the baby will descend against the cervix more easily during labor, which will help it wedge open faster.

The bottom line: A well positioned baby = a faster labor.

Assuming the position

Thanks to their beautiful big heads, human babies have really only one best way to fit through their mother's pelvis.

They need to turn upside down and face to the back of their moms, with their chins tucked to their chests. That gets the smallest diameter of the head, the crown, heading out first. Helpfully, about three weeks before their due date, most babies begin dropping of their own accord down into their mother's pelvis – a process that's called lightening. Ideally, they'll already be upside down and backwards by then. If their heads are a little cockeyed, labor can be much more painful and drawn out for mom.

What if the baby never turns?

If the baby refuses to turn at all or remains head up, it's in a breech position. Most doctors will try and turn it the right way up through hand manipulations (generally, between 36 and 38 weeks into the pregnancy. After 38 weeks, turning doesn't work so well and many doctors won't even try it). If turning doesn't work, you'll almost certainly be heading for a C-section as very few doctors will deliver a breeched baby vaginally any more (see our appendix on complications).

Helping the baby lighten

The good news is that mothers do have some control over optimal fetal positioning in the weeks prior to labor. They just need to use gravity and physics to their advantage.

The key, starting around four weeks before her due date, is for the mom to be very conscious of her posture.

As we'll explain, that's something you can both help with.

Let gravity do the work

For most people, this is mostly a matter of allowing gravity to help them out.

Remembering that the heaviest parts of a baby are the head and back, you want to allow the heavy side to swing forward and down. That allows the baby to be both upside down and facing the mother's spine.

Here's the way you'd like the baby to end up.

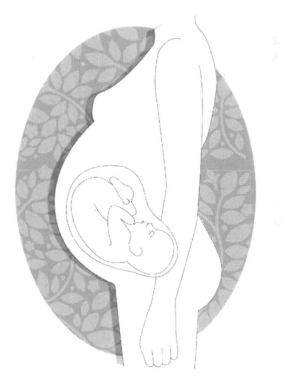

Facing backwards (anterior position)

Sometimes, though, the baby ends up like this.

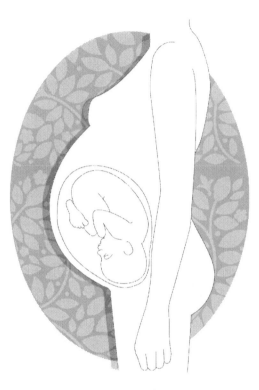

Facing forward (posterior position)

If that happens, there are a few things you can do to help the baby face in the optimal direction.

Sit up straight!

Pregnancy is exhausting and nothing seems more appropriate than encouraging the mom to spend a big chunk of it lounging on her comfy living room furniture. That's not so bad in the early months, but in the last four weeks, it's not going to help. Modern lounge furniture encourages slouching, unfortunately. What's much more helpful, though, is sitting up straight (just like your mother and grandmother told you!).

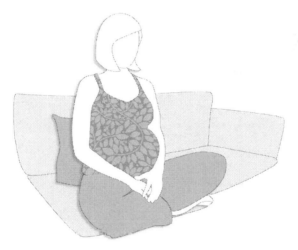

Couch sitting: Sit cross-legged as far back on the couch as possible with pillows supporting the low back

Of course, it's not particularly helpful if you slouch right next to her. You can at least sit up a bit straighter while she's doing the same—and it's good for your back, too!

Sitting on an exercise ball is a great alternative to a couch. It's still soft and supportive, but it forces the upright posture that we're looking for.

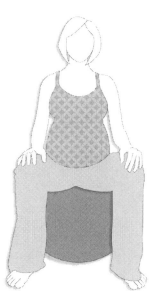

Sitting alternative: Sit on the front 1/3 of the ball with wide feet

Encourage your partner to use this positioning whenever she can – when watching TV, sitting at a desk, talking with friends.

If she's sitting on the floor, she can raise her bottom up on a couple of cushions and cross her legs, yoga-style. She should also have another cushion supporting her lower back.

It's also good idea for the mom-to-be to do some stretches on her hands and knees every day.

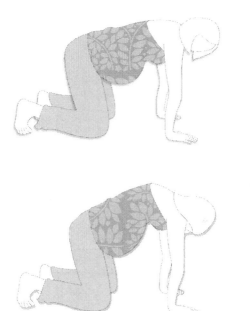

Stretch: Move from a flat back to a rounded back
(avoid arching your back)

Two more things to keep doing: walking and sex

Walking

If the mom's not having too much pelvic or back pain in the last month of pregnancy, it is a really good idea for her to get out and walk every day. Join her if you can.

This is one of the most important things she can do to make sure the baby is well positioned and that she doesn't go too far over its due date.

These do not need to be long walks. What you are looking for is for her to feel a sense of heaviness (it's great if she also feels her Braxton Hicks contractions a little more strongly) because that's a signal that the baby is dropping into the pelvis.

Love is the drug

As she nears her due date, sex may not be at the top of her list of things to do, but it is something you should both consider. Not only is it a loving thing in its own right, but sex can actually help facilitate labor.

This isn't so much about positioning – or physics – as chemistry. As her due date nears, a woman's body is already producing the hormones that will begin her labor. She can add to these hormones by making love.

Here are four ways in which sex has been found to help:
- Orgasm for the Woman: this produces oxytocin, which contracts the uterus
- Nipple Stimulation: this does the same thing
- Cuddling: ditto, again.
- Semen: contains prostaglandins that will help ripen a cervix.

A word of caution: *If her water has broken you don't want to put anything into the vagina. It can introduce bacteria that could cause an infection for her and the baby.*

But if her water hasn't broken and your medical caregiver confirms that there's nothing about the pregnancy that would contraindicate, sex is safe until the day she goes into labor.

Will sex hurt the baby?

Men can be nervous about hurting either their partner or the baby by having intercourse at this point, but she can tell you what is comfortable or not and the baby is well protected inside.

A woman shouldn't spend too much time on her back at this point in her pregnancy, because it's bad for her circulation, and she shouldn't have any heavy pressure on her abdomen. So, it's better to try sexual positions like spooning (side-to-side intercourse).

One other warning: don't blow into the vagina during oral sex. That can cause a rare but potentially fatal air embolus. You don't want that!

One for the team

It's totally understandable if sex, at this point, may not seem appealing to one or both of you. And, of course, that's okay. It may be time, though, to consider "taking one for the team." Sex, after all, is a really good way to keep her pregnancy from going far past her due date. Think about it. Talk about it. Give it a try, maybe.

If the thought is just more than one or both of you can bear, cuddling will also produce oxytocin. So spend some quality time snuggling on the couch each day and if you end up doing more than cuddling, then great!

BIRTH PLANS: A GOOD OR BAD IDEA?
CHAPTER FOUR

A birth plan is a written document that expresses the wishes of a couple for their labor, birth and immediate postpartum care.

Over the last few years birth plans have gotten something of a bad rap, perhaps with good reason.

After all, pretty much every birth has its unexpected twists and turns. They're simply not things that can be carefully planned out ahead of time, which is one reason why some doctors and nurses have come to see birth plans as pieces of wishful thinking that they can safely ignore.

Our position is a little different, though. When composed in the right spirit, we believe, birth plans can be extremely useful.

Women typically do have real options when giving birth – think: pain medication, for a start – which they have a right to voice and their caregivers have a duty to try and respect.

It's also worth recognizing that some common birthing practices (like hydrating women through IV tubes and thus restricting their movements) are rooted in a desire to make things convenient for the medical team and, arguably, a failure to appreciate how allowing a laboring woman to remain mobile can contribute to the likelihood of a fully natural, low-intervention birth. Which is both why and how birth plans become popular in the first place.

In addition, it's now pretty much established that a woman's state of mind can either hasten or impede the progress of her labor. It's just not a good idea to have a laboring mother feeling like she's not being heard.

A birth plan, then, can offer the mother both a way to communicate how she would like things to go and an easy vehicle through which everyone involved in her labor can get on board with those wishes.

Still, anyone writing a birth plan needs to recognize that it can't appear to ask doctors or nurses to go against their best medical judgment. And it needs to understand that even the best laid plans can – and in childbirth often do – need to be put aside to deal with what actually happens once the labor is underway.

From birth plans to birth preferences

Better, then to think of your birth plans as less about plans, per se, than preferences. They're there to express what you are hoping for. And that's a good thing to share.

So what should you hope for? It can be a whole bundle of things. We've seen birth plans that go on for pages. Those quickly become impossible to actually remember or keep track of, however, and they're understandably off-putting to the people trying to work with you in circumstances that can move quickly from slow and blissed-out to tense and fast-moving.

Instead, we recommend that you create a plan that is:
- Short – no longer than a page
- Written in a friendly, non-threatening tone
- Simple and clear – bullet points are great!

Writing the plan – first, research

Your plan should feature only the things that you and your partner really care about. So how do you decide what those are going to be?

For a start, you can think back to earlier births, if this isn't your first. Then talk to friends and, of course, to your trusted practitioners. If you've taken a birth class (see Chapter 2), you'll likely have a sense of the different preferences that women often have going into their labors. And think about where you plan to give birth – it will likely have its own standards and practices that you should be clear on before you make your plan.

You can also visit the 'Recommended' section of our website, www.deliverbook.com, which lists books, internet sites and web apps that you can consult at this point. And read the next chapter, about birth teams, and the one following, about pain medication. They will also help as you think about what you might want in your plan.

After you have educated yourself, you can begin jotting down things that are important to you. It's worth doing even if you end up deciding to leave the plan at home. Talking this through as a couple and getting yourself on the same page is the first step in forming a great birth team.

What to include

The most common preferences on birth plans cover three main topics:
- Your feelings about pain medication and pain management
- Your preferences on movement during labor and during the final, pushing stage.
- Your preferences for the baby immediately after birth

What else to include

The possibilities are alarmingly extensive, so read the list below while remembering that you need to keep your plan short. But it could mention that you'd like your partner to be able to:

Laboring options
- eat through labor if she can
- hydrate through drinking water or eating ice rather than through an IV
- allow nursing or medical students and other residents to be present (or not)
- keep the lights low during labor
- be able to play her own music or visualizations

- be free to walk around or use the shower or birthing tub
- be continuously monitored (or intermittently)
- have a private room, if available
- labor without time limits, if medically safe
- be free to use a video or still camera
- have intermittent fetal monitoring, if possible
- not have her waters broken artificially unless absolutely necessary
- not be induced without trying alternative measures (walking etc.) first
- have an epidural ASAP, or not at all
- prefer IV-delivered pain relief over an epidural
- not be offered pain relief unless she asks for it
- avoid an episiotomy if all possible
- determine her positions for pushing and delivery herself

Delivery options
- save the umbilical cord blood
- decide who cuts the cord
- take the placenta home with her, or view it
- be actively consulted in decisions relating to emergency caesarian deliveries
- allow birth partners to attend a caesarian birth

Newborn care options

- be able to breastfeed in the delivery room
- postpone any testing and vaccinations until after mother and child have had – a chance to bond
- have a son circumcised (or not) at the hospital
- have all newborn procedures done in her or her partner's presence
- waive certain standard procedures (such as administering eye drops, Vitamin K shot and bathing by someone other than you)

A sample plan

If all that leaves you feeling hopelessly overwhelmed, check out the appendix, where we have a sample birth pan that you're welcome to copy and adapt as you see fit.

FROM BIRTH PREFERENCES TO BIRTH TEAM

Where birth plans can get you into trouble is when they act as a barrier between the laboring mother and everyone else who is there to help her.

Assuming that you both have a plan that will help, not hinder, the team building that you need to do, let's think a bit more about who's on that team.

The core team of two

The first and most important members of the birth team are the two of you. We've already discussed how important it is for you both to talk openly about your hopes and fears surrounding the birth. But we'll say it again here: having one or more conversations about this, where you listen and learn about your partner's worries and concerns, will go a long way in making her labor day feel supported and satisfying.

While your fears and concerns are also important, you do need to remember that this is fundamentally about the person with the baby inside her. She's going to be doing the heavy lifting here, and because of that she gets to have the final say.

And partners, whether she is planning to do the whole thing *au naturale* or wants to have medication as soon you reach the hospital, you need to be prepared to watch her in some discomfort and pain. This can be a very hard thing to do. But if you are both clear on your feelings it can help.

Questions for the mom to answer are:
- Does she want pain medication?
- Does she want to go to the hospital as soon as possible or stay home for as long as she can, or something in between?
- Who else would she like to have there and how does she see those roles?
- What is she most nervous or afraid about?
- What specifically would she like from you?

Questions for her partner to answer are:
- How do you feel about the other people she wants with her?
- What role do you see for yourself and how does it differ from her view?
- Do you feel like you can do the things she wants?
- How do you feel about her stance on pain medication?
- Are you prepared to advocate and negotiate with hospital staff on her behalf?

Your answers to all of this can build into your plan. And having talked this through, you'll be on the same page.

Being there, or not

It's pretty much assumed these days that a child's father will be present at his children's birth. Little more than a generation ago, of course, that was not the case at all.

We're definitely in the camp that sees this change as a good thing. We believe that a) all men are capable of being fantastically supportive birth partners and b) they should be there to be that partner if they humanly can.

Still, for some couples, that's just not going to work. Because of the very particular personalities involved, or for religious or medical reasons (he has an infection, say), it's best that he not be there at the birth. If that's true in your case, your job is to be supportive right up to the point of labor and to ensure that your partner is getting the laboring support that she needs from someone else (a doula, say, or sister, or friend).

If your concern as a partner is more that you'll go to pieces, however, or that you're just a hopeless klutz, we understand. It's why we wrote the book, in some ways. In the course of just a few decades, men have gone from waiting outside the delivery room with flowers and a cigar at the ready, to being expected to attend births while offering near-professional-level support.

So we hear you. But we think that what's being asked of you is something you can totally do – especially if you take to heart the main points in this book.

Bottom line: All men can do a great job as labor supporters and, when they do that, they offer huge benefits to the laboring mom.

Add your doctor or midwife to the team

Now it's time for the pair of you to take your plan – and your confidence as a birth team – to the professionals.

A month or so before your due date, let your caregiver know that you'd like a few extra minutes at your next appointment to discuss your birth preferences and plan. As we suggested in the previous chapter, some caregivers may bristle at this, but you can explain to them that you trust their judgment and that you are just looking for clear communication while the stress is low.

They should appreciate, after all, that your foresight will make you more assured and calmer for the labor – which should only help them in their job, too. With luck, your discussion will make them more likely to take real note of your preferences and be flexible, within the realm of what they believe is safe for you and your baby.

Once your doctor or midwife has approved your birth plan, you now have a great tool to use with the final members of your birth team, your doula (if you choose to have one) and your labor and delivery nurses.

To doula or not

Of course, we have a personal bias toward hiring a doula since we've both used them with success and one of us is a doula. But we're also aware that, for various financial and personal reasons, doulas aren't for everyone. Still, we'd feel remiss if we didn't mention their numerous benefits. Throughout history, women have given birth surrounded by members of their family and/or local birth attendants – usually other women. This is not accidental. As you experience childbirth for the first time, there's a lot to be said for being in the presence of others who have a deep understanding of what that experience is like. And many recent scientific studies have born this out, showing that women who engage doulas experience multiple benefits. Among them:

- Shorter labors
- Less use of pain medication
- Fewer C-sections
- Greater satisfaction with birth and partner
- Feeling more bonded to baby
- Greater success with breastfeeding (up to six weeks postpartum)

So bringing a doula into the birth team is something that we believe that every couple should at least consider.

Your Labor and Delivery nurses – crucial strangers

Apart from each other, and your doula if you hire one, your labor and delivery nurses will be the people you'll see the most during your labor.

They're the final part of your birth team – but typically you won't meet any of them until the moment you arrive in the delivery ward (though with some midwifery groups and in the case of midwife-supervised home births, this won't be true).

Although we have another chapter to go before we get to the point where you meet them, we'll talk about how to communicate with them now, since working well with them will make a big difference to how your labor goes as a whole.

Remember, the doctor arrives late

While a few doctors still attend births from early in labor, the overwhelming majority only show up when the baby is very near to being born – unless there is a clear medical need to come earlier.

So, if you have gone the OB route, your nurses will be your main expert medical contacts for a substantial majority of the time you are in labor.

They also usually change shifts every 8 to 12 hours, so it is very likely that you will have more than one.

As we've already said, labor is a process that can be deeply impacted by the psychological state of the person going through it. Worry, upset, fear, and other kinds of free-floating unhappiness can all have a negative effect.

It is ironic, then, that the people with whom you'll be spending the vast majority of your time in labor will be complete strangers with whom you might instantly bond or fail ever to make a connection with.

Bonding with your nurses

The good news is that labor and delivery nurses are generally some of the most amazing people you'll ever meet. But, still, until she or he walks into the room, they won't know you from Adam.

So what can you do to make these important relationships work best for you and your partner – and fast?

1) Be friendly

Firstly, remember that nurses are professionals, and that everyone who comes into Labor and Delivery is nervous and needy (and rightly so).

Nurses are people, too, of course. Just like us, they have good and bad days – and the best thing you can do when you first meet them is to make an effort (however tired you are by now) to be friendly and try and make a connection with them right away.

Remember their name, perhaps, or compliment something (they often have their children's photos on the back of their ID badges around their necks). Maybe ask a simple question about them that doesn't have to do with their professional abilities. That will get you off to a great start.

2) Be cooperative (until you aren't)

For all the popular horror stories you hear of authoritarian or inconsiderate nurses, it's worth knowing that their patients are usually the ones who are more dictatorial or rude. Try, then, to start out being as cooperative as you can. Don't assume you need to go on the offense. Instead, go out of your way to be accommodating. Then when you make special requests later on, they won't see it as a pattern, but as a genuinely important desire.

3) Be considerate
Nurses have a lot of back office duties to take care of that you might not know about or see.

So when you arrive, for example, ask your nurses when would be a good time to share your birth plan with them. That alerts them to the fact that you have a plan but acknowledges that they don't need to see it right away and will be better able to really absorb it once they've done all the paperwork to check you in. When you give it to them, by the way, you should make mention that your doctor has already looked it over and approved it.

MEDICATION
CHAPTER SIX

Plenty of decisions about birth get made for you. A weak fetal heartbeat, or slow contractions, or a pinched umbilical cord – each will dictate that a specific set of procedures get put in motion.

But that's not true of everything, especially when it comes to the treatment of pain.

Medication – the biggest conundrum

Different people have different tolerances for pain. It's totally possible for a woman to endure great pain during labor, for example, and yet go entirely medication-free and afterwards feel nothing but positive about the experience.

Others, though, will have a great birth experience precisely because they accepted medication early in labor.

We vary, too, in being able to accurately predict how much pain we'll be able to handle when push comes to pushing even harder. Laboring mothers can be surprised both by how much and how little pain they turn out to be willing to endure. The woman who'd sworn she was having an epidural the minute she walks into the delivery room can find herself both willing and able to complete her labor drug-free. Or just the opposite can happen.

Because we can't always predict how things might change, it's a good idea if both of you already know some of the risks and benefits of pain medication before labor begins, so that you can help your partner make an informed choice for herself. It's also important for the birthing mom to cut herself some slack when she does go into labor and wants to change her plan. And it's just as important for her partner to support her, whatever she decides.

Support, whatever happens

That bears repeating: Whatever happens, it's your job to help her find the information she needs, work through it with her, and support her choice, even if it is not the one you would have made for yourself.

Again, that might mean going with Plan B. In that case, your job is to check that she's sure about changing the plan and then, if she is, support her 100%.

Equally, if she's determined to stick to her original plan – receiving only IV pain medication, for example – the last thing she needs is for her partner to keep offering her an epidural.

Remember, as we noted in chapter one, research tells us that women who feel like they've been heard during their labor:
- Feel a closer bond with their baby AND their partner
- Have less postpartum depression

- Are more likely to have successful breastfeeding experiences

The science of medication – the example of epidurals

Pain medication for labor and delivery has been massively researched but with annoyingly unclear results, especially when it comes to epidurals, the most potent form of birth-related pain control. You can pretty much find a study on epidurals that will tell you whatever it is about them that you want to hear. Some suggest that epidurals lengthen labor, for example, while others say they shorten it. We've seen them do both.

What is true is that an epidural has a lot of paraphernalia that goes with it. With an epidural, the mother is confined to bed for remainder of her labor, will need an IV, a blood pressure cuff and a bladder catheter. Epidurals also make it more likely that the mother will need a drug like Pitocin to keep her labor moving along, as well as other medications for blood pressure, itching or nausea.

There is an upside, though, of course: thanks to the epidural, her pain will be greatly decreased or even completely eliminated.

Again, the key thing here is to get informed. Do more reading, and quiz your doctor and your childbirth educators about your options and then make a plan for how you'd like to proceed, always knowing that plans can change.

The same goes for any and all choices surrounding pain management in labor.

Rules for partners, whatever her choices

No matter what the laboring woman's preferences, there are some basic guidelines that partners can usefully follow:

1) **Don't offer her pain medication.** Even if she looks really uncomfortable, let her ask for it. She won't have forgotten that pain medication is available and, despite her discomfort, she may be feeling like she's doing great until you suggest otherwise. Women in labor are highly suggestible. Tell her she is doing great and she'll likely agree.

2) **Make a plan for talking about Plan B.** If she's trying to avoid medication, it's a good idea to talk about what you will do to support her if she begins talking about medication or asks for it. It's best to do this in advance and with your doula (if you have one) and other medical care givers at a prenatal visit. One option that works well is to not bring up pain medication at all, and instead give lots of encouragement and suggestions to distract (we'll go into this more in Chapter 7). If she begins say that she thinks she won't make it, you can plan to then increase your encouragement and support – she hasn't asked for medication yet, after all.

3) **Try and hold off pain meds, at least at first.** Waiting until labor is well established and a woman is dilated to 4 or 5 centimeters has been shown to help avoid unwanted complications and interventions. This isn't always possible, for sure. Sometimes a woman will be in very hard, painful labor

before she gets to that stage. But it's worth knowing that in an "average" labor, most women can make it to 4 or 5 centimeters simply with good support.

4) **You don't need to overdo things.** If your partner has an epidural, be aware that it can be too numbing. Once it's in place, she should not feel any pain but she should feel some pressure sensations. If she has no sense at all that she is having contractions and can't move her legs, the epidural is probably heavier than it needs to be and runs a risk of interfering and slowing down the labor. Be sure you speak with the anesthesiologist about this so it can be adjusted.

5) **Think about turning it down at the end.** When it is time to begin pushing (see chapter 10), if her epidural feels very heavy and she is not feeling any pressure with contractions, it is a good idea to ask for the epidural to be turned down now. Not off, just down. This allows for her to push more effectively and will hopefully speed the along the baby's birth.

Again, there is no "right" way to have your baby.

Bottom line: your job is to help your partner to make the decisions that she believes are right for her without feeling pressured or disempowered by friends, family and/or medical personnel.

More tips for helping avoid an epidural

If that's what she wants, here's a way to try and help her get there, even when she's having a really hard time with the pain:

First as we mentioned above, don't talk about pain medication before she does, because if she hasn't actually asked for it, she's likely doing okay. But the truth is that women also often just want to vent. Just because she's complaining loudly, then, you don't need to jump ahead and assume that she's asking for an epidural.

If she continues complaining and becomes increasingly vocal about it or if she actually asks for medication, you can set a time frame. Suggest that she get in the shower, perhaps, or change position, for prescribed length of time (20 minutes often feels doable). At the end of that time, you can ask the nurse to check her progress and then make a decision. If she is dilated to 8 or 9 cm, you can remind her that it will be a very short time until she is pushing. If she is at 3 or 4, she might feel that she is done and needs some relief.

In either case, planning for this approach beforehand can helps you both be a little more sure during the heat of the labor that her wishes are being followed. Remember, she is going to say it hurts, and that she is tired and that this sucks. All of that is true, because that's how labor feels without medication. But none of it is a call for medication either, and many, many women come out the other end finding that they never actually asked for it and very glad they didn't. So let her be the one to ask.

EARLY LABOR:
SHE'S CONTRACTING, SO YOU'RE DISTRACTING
CHAPTER SEVEN

A while back, your partner's doctor will have given her a list of reasons to call outside of her usual appointment schedule. It will cover concerns such as bleeding, fevers, pain, swelling or trauma to the abdomen and more. And naturally, if anything on that list occurs, she'll contact her OB right away.

But its much more likely that you'll both be wondering why nothing seems to be happening at all. In the last few weeks, it really can seem like the final onset of labor will never arrive. At some point, though, your partner will go into labor.

Your medical experts might not want to wait, of course. For a variety of reasons they might want to induce her labor, or perform a Cesarean, both of which we'll look at in our appendix on complications.

But that's not typical. Much more often, a women goes into labor of her own accord.

What does it mean for labor to start?

Essentially, her Braxton Hicks contractions start getting both more frequent and more intense.

In the days and hours leading up to 'real' labor you might see:
- Losing the mucous plug from the vagina
- Spotting (little bits of blood)
- Loose stool and stomach upset
- Nesting (a new and distinct urge to clean, tidy and organize)
- Increased Braxton Hicks

Officially, real labor begins when;
- Her waters have broken

or
- When her contractions have begun to form a pattern of short intervals of discomfort followed by feeling fine – and when those intervals start getting stronger, longer and closer together.

That's both exciting and daunting.

It means that you'll meet your baby really soon. But it also means that your partner now faces the most intense and uncertain part of her pregnancy.

No wonder, then, that the question we get asked most about this stage is: what can we do to make this stage go swiftly and painlessly?

Certainly, even if things go perfectly, no labor will ever be a walk in the park. But there is a fair amount that a mom – and her partner – can do to make her labor feel both shorter and less uncomfortable, particularly in the early stages.

Having a strategy - or, ignorance is bliss

Here's one very simple way to make it feel shorter: Ignore the early part.

Most first-time parents make the mistake of being hyperaware of her every contraction right from the start, carefully logging and timing the length of each and every one. Expectant dads are particularly guilty of this!

Early on, though, it just isn't necessary. Get a rough idea of how fast her contractions are coming and how long they're lasting – then relax. Doing much more in the early stages only stresses the mom out, which can quickly wear her out, too. It helps to remember that the longest part of labor is usually the time it takes to get the cervix dilated to three centimeters. That typically lasts 6-8 hours for first-timers, but it can be much longer.

In most cases, you really need to do this at home. Go to the hospital at this point, and the staff is almost certain to send you straight back.

But her contractions have started. They're tight, involuntary muscle spasms that are both exciting and little scary to experience. Still, they aren't what you could describe as overwhelming – yet.

Right now they're likely to be spread out (5-20 minutes apart) and short (under a minute). That spacing, coupled with their relatively mild intensity, means they're pretty manageable at present, especially with your help. Think of it like this: if her contractions are 15 minutes apart and 30 seconds long, for how much of any hour is she uncomfortable? That's right, just two minutes. So don't sit around worrying and waiting for those two minutes for the whole rest of the hour!

How do you stop yourselves from doing that? This is where you, the birth partner, really come into your own : it's your job right now to offer her loving distractions.

What you do depends on the time of day

If your partner begins contracting near bedtime, a great thing for her to do is to just take a bath and go to bed. And you too. Get out the candles, the mellow music, the aromatherapy thingy that's been sitting in the closet for the last year and a half. All of that's great too. Just don't make a great performance of it. Enjoy. Relax. Then go to bed. It's highly unlikely that either of you will miss anything – we can pretty much guarantee that no woman is going to sleep through the end stages of labor!

In fact, a sign that it is time to think about going to the hospital is when she can't tolerate being in bed during contractions anymore. But we can't stress enough how important it is to not stay up all night timing contractions down to the second when they are still sporadic.
Yes, you're both excited. Yes, you have a cool smart phone application for contraction timing, but right now you both need to rest.

Pretty much the same thing applies if your partner wakes up before morning with early labor contractions. She should stay in bed if she can. She'll probably doze in between the contractions. And even if she doesn't, just being horizontal is restful and that rest will be crucial later.

If her labor starts during waking hours

Once she's woken up from that night of light contractions interspersed with snoozing – or if labor begins during the day – here's what you can do: alternate activity with rest.

Activities could be:
- Going for a walk
- Going shopping
- Going out to eat

Resting could mean:
- Watching a movie
- Giving her a massage
- Having her take a bath or shower (sure, you can join in)

Here are some restful positions:

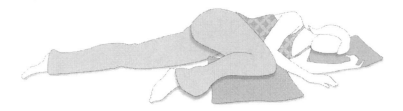

The Texas Roll: Top leg bent on pillow with bottom leg straight

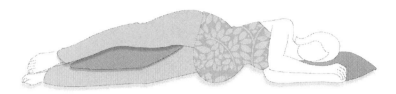

Side Resting: Pillow between the knee

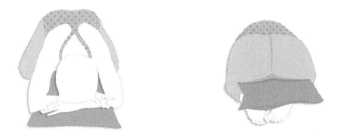

Child's pose: Toes together, knees apart for belly space.
Pillow between heels and bottom

Her activity and changing positions will help open her pelvis. That will move the baby down and stimulate further contractions – in other words, progress the labor.

The resting serves the important purpose of conserving energy and helping her to relax.

Hormones to watch out for – one good, one bad

As you'll both well know by now, pregnancy is all about hormones coursing through her body in powerful combinations for a full 9 months (and more). But two hormones in particular are very important during labor. One needs to be avoided and the other encouraged.

Adrenalin: the anti-labor hormone

Our bodies release adrenalin in stressful situations to give us the speed and energy to fight or take flight. Unfortunately a woman does neither of these things with her uterus. When a woman is stressed during labor, her body takes energy and focus away from her contractions. So get her more worried, worked up or scared than she already is and you slow down her labor. That, in turn, can make the whole thing seem more painful that it otherwise would. Indeed, your job is to do just the opposite.

Oxytocin: hormone of love

Oxytocin, on the other hand, is what she wants lots of. It's produced when we feel love, have an orgasm, eat chocolate – or come across many other pleasing situations. Crucially, it also causes the uterus to contract, so it needs to be encouraged throughout a woman's labor.

When you think about it, this is very cool: doing everything that makes a woman feel pampered and really loved will, rather wonderfully, also speed her labor and make it feel less bad.

Inducing oxytocin – your emphasis is on love

Birth partners have something else on their side here: activities that produce Oxytocin also help reduce Adrenalin production.

Any of these should help stimulate the good stuff and reduce the bad:

- Doing some relaxing breathing together
- Listening to music that stirs happy memories
- Watching a romantic comedy
- Visualizing a happy scene or place
- Giving her a foot rub
- Eating a little chocolate
- Cuddling together

Want to up the ante for a labor that feels slow?

- Give her an orgasm (but without intercourse if her waters have broken)
- Stimulate her nipples

Now, if you suggest the sex thing and she says, 'Are you kidding?' don't push it. That's not romantic and will get the wrong hormone flowing. But otherwise, this is another pre-birth win-win.

The stomach factor – don't forget to feed her

Here's the rule on food and labor: If a woman's hungry, feed her.

For many years, food was restricted for laboring women to reduce the chance of aspiration (choking) in the rare cases that she'd go on to need general anesthesia. Modern recommendations and research by the World Health Organization, however, suggest that this practice is not beneficial and can actually be harmful.

Why? Because labor amounts to a monster workout, which takes a lot of energy.

So laboring women, especially in the early stage, should eat frequent light meals and snacks for as long as they want them. Let her tastes lead you, but a good rule of thumb is to offer her things that are easy to digest (soup and smoothies, for example), have some protein in them for staying power (scrambled eggs, yogurt) and that you don't mind seeing again (yes, vomiting might happen).

Staying hydrated – sip, sip, and then sip a little more

When you are dehydrated, your muscles are weak and inefficient. And the uterus, remember, is a large muscle. If a woman gets dehydrated in labor she'll have frequent, painful contractions that don't open her cervix. Neither of you want her to go there.

You can easily help avoid what the pro's call 'pain with no purpose' by encouraging her to take frequent sips of water, juice, or Gatorade throughout.

Bottom line: make sure that she's remembering to pee often. You don't have to be the one to check the color, but you could gently remind her that it would be a good idea for someone to look and that if her pee's anything other than light yellow or clear, she needs to up the amount of fluid that she's taking in.

When to go to the hospital – seriously, there's no rush

It's probably the biggest worry of all in early-stage labor: What if we leave it too late?

Movie directors love that scene where the parents-to-be make a mad dash for the hospital and it's too late and dad has to deliver the baby in the taxi cab.

But really, for nearly all first time parents, the danger is just the opposite: that they'll go to the hospital too soon. Do that, and you'll be there for hours that you could as easily – and more comfortably – have spent at home. And that's the best case scenario. More likely, you'll get sent home and told to come back later, which can be both disheartening and frustrating for the mother (i.e., not good for Oxytocin).

Of course, all laboring couples are eager to get to the place where their baby will be born so they can hunker down and feel ready.

But the truth is that most people will feel more relaxed, and thus labor better, at home. The hospital and the trip there can also raise adrenalin (i.e., help inhibit labor), so it's really worth trying to stay home as long as you feel able. In fact, some of our favorite OBs say that the best way to avoid medical interventions in childbirth is for the laboring mother to stay out of the hospital for as long as she possibly can.

But how do you know it is time? – defining 'active'

A woman is usually admitted to hospital when she is in 'active labor' and 3-4 centimeters dilated. You probably won't be doing cervical checks at home, though. So how will you know? Though every woman and every labor is different, here are some signs that active labor has begun:

- Her breathing with contractions becomes heavier
- She needs to focus during contractions
- She loses her sense of humor
- She can no longer walk and talk through contractions/ wants to lean during them
- She doesn't want to sit or lie down with contractions
- She feels nauseated or vomits
- She has 5-1-1 contractions: i.e. she has contractions that are 5 minutes or less apart, that last for at least 1 minute, over a period of at least 1 hour

If your mom-to-be is exhibiting most of these signs, she's probably in active labor.

How to time contractions

Contractions are timed from the beginning of one contraction until the beginning of the next, so the length of a contraction is included when you are figuring out how far apart they are. If you have a contraction that is one minute long and it was four minutes between the end of one and the beginning of the next you would say they were five minutes apart and lasting one minute.

You want to note both how long contractions are and how far they are apart when you are thinking about when to go to the hospital or calling your midwife if you are having the birth at home.

Your job is counting

For her, it's all about the contractions now. They've become the only thing she's thinking about.

For guys, this is the time to whip out that contraction-counting application or a good old-fashioned watch (see above for how to count). This will give you a solid handle on what's actually happening – as opposed to what, in your excitement, you might think is going on.

But remember, there's still probably no rush. Active labor generally averages 2-5 hours and the next two stages – transition and pushing – usually last another 2-4 together. When you have decided it really is time to go, in other words, you can be still relaxed and calm about it (and therefore continuing to help the baby along).

If in doubt, obviously, you can call your OB. But he or she won't be wanting to get to the hospital any earlier than necessary, either.

What to take to the hospital – a dad's pack list

There's a whole industry devoted to listing (and selling) all the items an expectant mom is supposed to take with her to the hospital. We've even got our own list in the back of the book, but here are some things you might pack for yourself:
- Gum or mints
- Toothbrush and toothpaste
- Warm sweatshirt (hospitals are cold and women run hot)
- Hot water bottle (for lower back or anywhere that's sore)

- Snacks
- A book or magazines (for when she's reading)
- Your address book (if it's not in your phone)
- Your mobile phone
- Massage lotion
- A massage tool for when your hands get tired
- A surprise comfort object for mom (a soft blanket, favorite slippers, a religious medallion/rosary/hand of God – you know her best)

When to rush

Whatever we say about most babies taking a long time to arrive, some little ones, of course, are in a hurry to be born. If you suddenly find the following things happening, you need to get to the hospital as quickly as you can:
- Contractions are three minutes or less apart
- Contractions are a minute or more long
- She's feeling like she needs to poop but can't (it may be the baby's head!)

Even if you do notice these signs and decide to leave right away, rest assured that with first babies, you still likely have plenty of time to make the trip.

ACTIVE LABOR:
COMFORT AND CHEER(LEADING)
CHAPTER EIGHT

You're now in the place where your baby will be born.

Most likely, you're in a hospital, in the part designed to do nothing but help babies come safely into the world. Congratulations!

Unfortunately, though, many Labor and Delivery rooms aren't designed to be comfortable or relaxing for laboring mothers-to-be. That's not so good, because her comfort really matters right now.

Making her comfortable in an uncomfortable place

Being in a hospital usually means that something's wrong either with us or with someone we love. So it's not uncommon for a woman to feel, just by being there, that something must be wrong either with her or the baby, when that's nothing like the case.

Remember the laboring mom's nemesis, adrenalin? Just being in a hospital can produce that labor-slowing hormone. Luckily, though, she has you – and this is a situation you can do a fair bit to change.

Here's how you can make a hospital environment a little more homey and relaxing:
- Dim the lights (bright florescents feel like a spotlight on a laboring woman)
- Play music to create a space that belongs to you (see our playlist suggestions at www.deliverbook.com)
- Show her photos of people and things she loves (that's why you bought your phone right? So pre-load it up with cute pictures she's not seen before. She'll love it.)
- Pull out that surprise comfort object for her you brought for her (see our 'Dad Pack' ideas)
- Get that nice smelling lotion out of the pack and give her a massage

Most of these assume you've brought your 'Dad's Pack' with you. If you skipped the last chapter, go back and check what you can bring. If you're in the hospital reading this for the first time on your iPad or Kindle, don't panic – you can still dim the lights and go beg some skin lotion. Then you can get started on the rub.

If you are planning to have your birth at home, you'll have all this taken care of well before she's gone into labor, right? Right.

Time to get out the birth plan

It's not a bad idea to post your plan right away on the outside door of the delivery room, so do that now. Sure, you don't want to be one of 'those' parents, but OBs have told us that otherwise they'll walk in the room and they won't know exactly what the patients want.

The same goes for nurses, who change over every few hours, remember. Getting the plan up in an easily spotted place can save you having to explain your preferences over again later on – again, if your plan is reasonable and you share it, you can expect it to be honored.

The big rub – at this point, better than sex

Touch is crucial to the health of everyone, young and old. And it is one of the best ways to comfort a laboring woman. Many men are nervous about it, though. They worry they'll be yelled at if they get it wrong and make a tense situation worse, so they often hold back. Here's our advice, though: just do it. Okay, you may get told to stop something you are trying and it may not always be in her most considered and temperate voice, but believe us, it is a rare woman who won't find any comfort at all in a massage. You just have to keep going until you find something that works.

Here are some simple but powerful techniques to try during contractions, or in between.

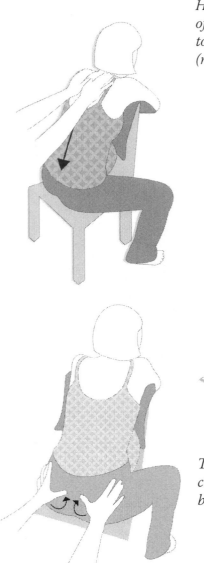

Heavy hands: With the flat of the hand, slowly drag from top to bottom at a steady pace (repeat)

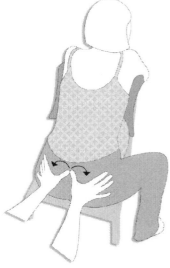

Thumb circles: Make large circles on the lower back, below the waistband.

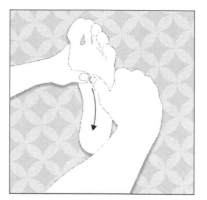

*Long strokes down the entire arch, firm pressure below
the ball of the foot*

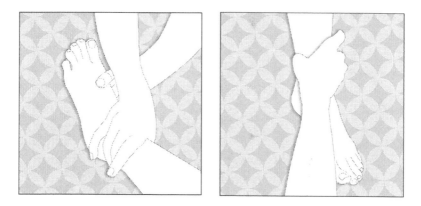

*Ankle squeeze:
Circle fingers around ankle just above the ankle bone with
thumbs pressing into the Achilles tendon.*

The secret to massage – mean it

If all these diagrams are way more than you can handle, you really only have to remember this one thing: massage is all about the intention. Truly, that's it. All you really need to do in order give someone a decent massage is to mean it.

When you are touching her, really be there, trying to comfort her. Want to help her and you will.

Inhale, exhale, repeat – breathing lessons

How else can you help? Breathing is perhaps the biggest area.

Remember, that exaggerated panting-thing sitcoms love to trot out when they show someone about to give birth? You likely tried it in a birthing class yourself and felt pretty stupid. But at this point in a labor, heavy breathing will be her – and your – best friend.

Breathing, of course, is something we do all the time without even thinking, but it's also is one of the most powerful labor comfort techniques there is.

Here's why: When we are in pain or under stress, our natural reaction is to hold our breath. But that's just what a mom should not be doing right now. Instead, she wants to keep her breath flowing. That does several important things.
It:

- Keeps mom and baby oxygenated
- Relaxes and lowers blood pressure and adrenalin
- Is a focal point that can distract from the pain of

contractions
- Provides energy and strength for all muscles including the uterus
- Helps her access power, both physical and mental

Breathing 101:

Most women can get through the lion's share of labor with one simple breathing technique. Amazing but true.
- Breath in deeply through the nose
- Breath out smoothly through the mouth
- Keep noises (that will come) low and open rather than high and tight.
- Repeat
- Repeat
- Repeat some more

Oh, the baby! - assuming the position/s.

The good thing about being in a hospital (or at home with a midwife) is that someone else is there whose job it is to worry about the safety of baby as well as the mom. That means you can focus on mom.

But what you are all there for, of course, is to work together to deliver a baby as naturally, safely and quickly as you can. How the mom lies or sits makes a big difference here, so it's worth keeping that in mind.

The average laboring woman will need to keep moving between several different positions throughout her labor.

Staying in any one position for a long time becomes incredibly uncomfortable. Switching positions helps break up the time as well. But most crucially, it also helps move the baby down through the pelvis.

You can help here by having one or two positions in mind at all times, ready to suggest another when it's clear she needs to change but is out of inspiration.

Here are some laboring positions to choose from:

Slow dancing: hold her under the arms to help support her weight, if needed; wide feet, sway gently

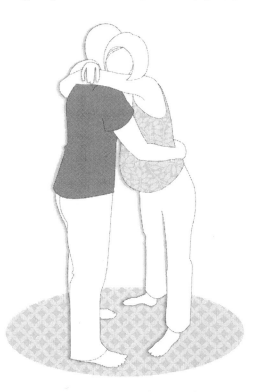

Lunge: place one foot on stable object, lean in and out

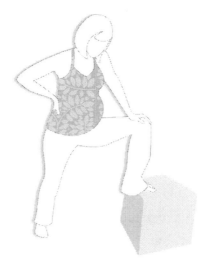

Hands and knees on floor or bed; helps with back pain

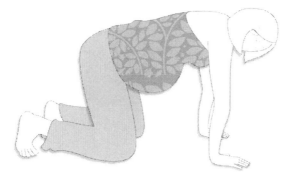

Child's pose: toes together, knees apart.
Restful if lying on side hurts.

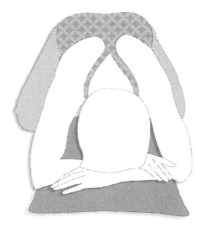

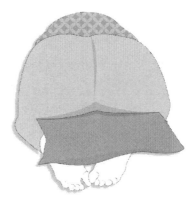

The birth ball: Will you actually ever use that thing?

You might. Many hospitals now have birth balls ('exercise balls' for those of us who aren't in labor), so check to see if yours does and, if they don't, try and bring one with you.

Remember, delivery rooms are generally short of comfortable alternative rest spots, and these big inflatables really expand her choice of positions that are both comfortable and also help move the baby down.

Ball and knees: Drape body over to rest between and during contractions

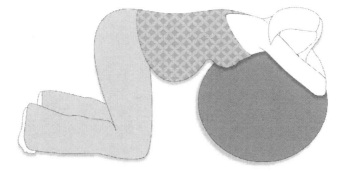

Sit on ball and gently roll in circles to open pelvis

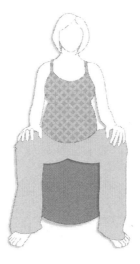

Other comforting ideas – like getting wet

Hydrotherapy is a fancy name for the fact that water makes humans feel better.

Warm water, either in a shower or a deep bath (so long as her membrane is intact), helps a laboring woman relax and experience her contractions as milder. Indeed, water can work near miracles in labor. It's why a lot of women choose water births, after all.

When in doubt – or a rut, or because you're both tired and bored and looking for a change – suggest water.

It's not uncommon for laboring moms to get in and out of the shower many times over the period of her labor. That's great. Again, it helps break up the time and gives her something to do, and moving in and out of the shower helps the baby move on down.

Once in there, try focusing the spray on her lower back or belly during contractions.

It's worth remembering that it can be hard to get a laboring woman to change positions. Even if you both are pretty convinced that getting in the shower (or getting out of bed to walk a little) is going to be a big help, it may take confident, loving and repeated encouragement to make the shift.

Visualization - sweet-talking her though

Labor can go on for a long, long time. That's usually perfectly okay for the baby, but it can be really, really draining on the mom.

As time goes on, even if things are progressing, she can get downhearted. If she gets really down, she can stop making progress and need medical intervention, which carries a whole new set of risks. You can help forestall this by employing a simple, safe tool: your voice.

If you see her starting to get drained and pessimistic, talk to her. Take her off to another mental place. It can make her feel less alone and actually help progress her labor.

Visualization ideas – you talk, it helps

There are three basic types you can try:

Process: "Your cervix is melting open" "The baby is moving down" "Dive into the center of this wave and let it flow over you."

End Game: "Pretty soon we'll be holding our daughter" "One year from now we will be having her birthday. Think how excited she will be with the cake."

Happy Place: "Remember that beach we spent so much time at on our honeymoon?" (describe it). "Remember that restaurant I took you to on our first date?" (then elaborate)

Try different kinds of visualizations as you feel like they might be helpful. Keep your voice smooth, rhythmic, relaxed. Hearing you will make her feel calmer.

BIRTH EMOTIONS
CHAPTER NINE

Here's another cliché of childbirth that has its basis in truth: There will probably be times, especially in an un-medicated labor, where the woman you love will become a stranger to you.

That's just the way it is. It's not bad. It's no reflection on you. You're both on journeys here and you'll both end up in the same place. But she'll be taking a totally different, and incredibly intense, route to get there.

Here are some normal emotions that she'll typically experience, starting with early labor:
- Excitement
- Nervousness
- Impatience
- Becoming inwardly focused during contractions
- Needing support, susceptible to suggestions, both encouraging and discouraging
- Facing self-doubt and feeling defeated

During labor, this woman whom you know better than anyone in the room will make sounds you have never heard. At times, she'll seem disoriented. There will be moments when, looking at her, you'll be sure something is very wrong.

Usually, though, the truth is quite the opposite. She's acting just as a laboring woman does – and should – act.

If you are worried, of course, call or ask a medical professional to check that she's okay. This will help you be even more confident when you assure her (as you need to, over and over) that she is doing great, that she is strong and that everything is perfect.

She needs encouragement

That's what she needs most from you right now, even when she hardly seems to know who's sitting there with her. It's so important we can't emphasize it enough: Laboring women cannot ever, ever hear enough encouragement. And that's your job!

Birth emotions – you are the rock

You, too, are also going to be running an emotional marathon.

For one thing, it's hard to see someone you love working so hard and being so uncomfortable and not being able to fix it. But try to remember that you can't fix it and you are not supposed to. You can, though, make her experience a whole heck of a lot better, which is what you've been doing so well so far.

But what if you are getting freaked out here, too? Well, the answer's simple if not particularly sympathetic: you've got to get over it.

Under normal circumstances we'd never recommend this, but right now you need to shelve whatever negative emotions you may be feeling. Right now, you get to be The Rock. That's right: unwavering in your support, unbowed in your optimism, absolutely certain of your confidence in her.

Here's the thing: at this point she will be taking a lot of cues from everyone around her. Doctors and nurses know that. They'll be wearing their game faces right now. You should have yours on too. You need to be a calm, encouraging mirror for her.

At this moment, that's your biggest job. And you can do it, because thousands of men do it every day.

You can tell her later about how you were really feeling. It's going to be a great story to share one day. But not now.

Take care of yourself

Just to be clear, though: we're not suggesting you have to be a martyr to the mother and child. You need to take care of yourself as well. You won't be any help to anyone if you are fainting, falling asleep or otherwise rapidly fading out of the picture.

Make sure you are eating and drinking. Grab a catnap in early labor when she does the same. And if you need to step out to collect yourself when things get really intense, go ahead and take five. Only make sure she's not alone before you do and come back soon – she needs you.

Here comes baby! - how to tell that you're getting close

It will happen. Really, it will. Somehow that baby will come out. And by this point you are very nearly there.

But how will you know if it's getting close to that time? The nurse, midwife or doctor, of course, might be in the room and just tell you. But they aren't going to be with you the whole time – even during some of her most intense contractions (so be ready for that!).

Here, then, are some reliable signs you can watch for to know that the baby is about to arrive:
- Contractions that are very close together and hard
- The mom starts doubting herself and wanting to quit
- Increased bloody discharge
- Rectal pressure – she feels like she needs to poop but can't
- Nausea
- Involuntary shaking
- Hot flashes and chills

If she's experiencing several of these things together, it's time to get the nurse in to check her.

The best thing is that these are all GOOD signs. Most likely, she's close to being able to push.

If she has an epidural - you're still needed

Most woman experience a dramatic shift once pain medication is administered. If it's done well and the pain is removed, she will be a lot more like the woman you're familiar with.

As less of her attention is focused on managing pain, she may feel less afraid and more relaxed. This can be just what was needed, especially when a labor has been prolonged or where the pain is creating so much fear and tension that it's impeding her progress.

After working so hard to support her, it can feel like your job is done once she gets an epidural. But this really isn't the time to pull out your laptop and catch up on email. If she sleeps, which is probably one of the best things for her to do, you should try to get some rest as well. You both have some seriously sleepless nights in your near future, after all!

If she is awake, pull your chair close to her bed, hold her hand, stroke her hair and talk, if she would like. Read to her from a magazine. Be together. She will still have anxiety about things to come and knowing that you are really there with her can make all the difference.

PUSHING THROUGH TO BIRTH
CHAPTER TEN

What's next – usually called 'Second Stage' or 'pushing and delivery' – can feel like a totally different ballgame.

In the first stage of labor, you were helping your partner manage her contractions as best she could while her cervix dilated. A lot of that was about waiting. In second stage, women have a much more active role. They can now begin to add their strength and force to the contractions and how much longer they have to go starts to become related to how hard they push.

This is where all that yoga and your helpful efforts to keep her relaxed, fed, hydrated, etc., up to this point will really pay off.

When is Second Stage?

Two things need to be in place before a woman can effectively start pushing. First, her cervix needs to be completely dilated, which it is at a diameter of roughly 10 cm. It's not uncommon for women to feel the urge to push before that, but that's usually not useful and could even cause the cervix to swell, which effectively reverses progress a bit. If she is feeling that urge to push early, you can help her pant through contractions and take positions that use gravity to her advantage (i.e., supporting herself face down on her forearms and knees with her bottom in the air).

Second, it's best to wait to begin pushing until the mom feels the urge to do so. Women can sometimes be completely dilated and still not want to push for 20 minutes or so. If a woman is un-medicated, this feeling is usually undeniable and feels like a really huge bowel movement (it's that romantic!), but even with an epidural a woman should begin to feel a heavy feeling in her bottom with contractions so that she will be able to push effectively and not spend too much energy with unproductive effort.

Positions: getting the cork out of the bottle

Just as in the early part of labor, changing positions can speed things along, helping the baby to move through the pelvis. Again, adding gravity to the equation is almost always helpful.

If you are in the hospital, the default pushing position is typically with her on her back with her knees up by her ears, just like on TV. But she has other options, all of which are variations on a basic squat.

Hands and knees

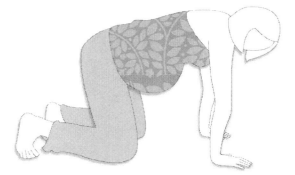

Side lying, holding onto leg for traction

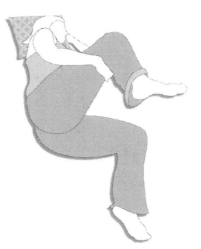

Squatting: Pelvic outlet is larger than when she is on her back

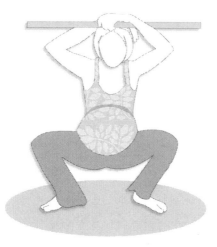

You have to be in a "squat" to deliver a baby. If you think about it, even lying on your back is a squat of sorts, just not one that utilizes gravity. But your squat can just as easily be upright, on your side, on your back, or on hands and knees – that's how the pelvis needs to be configured to get the baby out.

Remember, for first time moms the average pushing time is around two hours (it's typically much faster for second timers). So she has time to change positions every half hour or so and that can assist the baby to move down and out.

Breathing: Holding her breath vs. spontaneous bearing down

There's a surprising amount of debate about the best way to breath during pushing.

In hospital, they will usually direct a laboring mother to take a big breath when she starts the contraction and then bear down as if she's pooping while holding her breath. This can be very effective in getting babies out, particularly when a woman has an epidural and may not be feeling as much sensation to guide her and has less muscle control and power.

If that's is not working for her, though, or if it feels uncomfortable, she feels dizzy or the baby seems to be struggling according to the monitor, it is a good idea for her to try and follow her own urges.

This is called spontaneous bearing down. It is something that most of us do every day when we have a bowel movement. We feel like we have to go, take a breath, hold it for a few seconds while we brace our abdominal muscles and exhale (perhaps even grunt a little) as we push.

Ramp that up to the nth degree and you have what it takes to get a baby out. In the end, though, neither way is wrong. There is just the way that works for her.

What you will see at birth:

As she is pushing, you will be seeing her making Herculean efforts and it can be a little worrisome that in the beginning you don't see any results externally. Internally lots is going on, though.

The baby's head is being molded by the bony structures that surrouded the birth canal, the mom's tissues are stretching, and her pelvis is shifting.

After a while you will see some bulging in her perineum and then the labia will open with pushes and you'll begin to see just the tip of the head. In between pushes this progress can disappear, but remember that with each push she brings the baby down to where it was in the last push and then a little more. As more and more of the head emerges, the baby will crown, which means that the top of the head is visible.

From here on, things start to move fast.

The rest of the head and shoulders will usually emerge with just one more contraction and then, suddenly, a child has joined the world. A brand new person who will change your entire life.

You have a baby! Now what?

There are plenty of great books that rehearse all the details of the procedures typically followed immediately after birth, and they are fascinating (at least to us), but let's cut to the chase.

Ideally, what happens next is that baby goes right onto mom with skin-to-skin contact. If mom is wearing something, it should be lifted to let the baby touch her skin – that squirming slippery baby goes right there on her belly and breasts. The nurses can dry the baby to keep it from losing body heat and then cover mom and babe with a warm, dry blanket.

All the procedures that need to be done in a normal, non-eventful delivery can be done while mom holds the baby and you both get to know your new little one. Assigning Apgar scores, clearing breathing passages with a bulb syringe, listening to the heartbeat, cutting the cord, can all done while baby is being cradled by the mom.

This may or may not be what your medical team are used to or what's most convenient for them. So if you and your partner want this to happen, you might need to have already articulated it as part of your birth plan – and you might have to remind everyone of what your preferences are again at this point. Again, if there's a medically urgent reason to do otherwise, of course, that's what you do.

The typical alternative is to put the child on a 'warming table' somewhere across the room. Advantages to mom and baby of their cuddling instead of using the warming table abound. Here are just a few:

- Better maintenance of baby's body temperature
- Better bonding between mom and baby
- Baby calms down more quickly
- Better initiation of breastfeeding
- Cuter photos

During this time the doctor will be delivering the placenta, checking for bleeding and doing any suturing that is needed to the mom's perineum.

One last important word

Don't forget to initiate breastfeeding as soon as possible if you can (within that first hour).

When the baby starts making mouthing and rooting motions and mom has "caught her breath" from the delivery, breastfeeding should be started. That helps everything from slowing bleeding, to starting milk supply, to bonding.

The nurses can often help with getting mom and baby in a comfortable position, or, if you've taken a breastfeeding class together, you can help.

Your advocacy can be really helpful at this point.

Yes, there may be a good medical reason to have mom and baby separated at this point. But if there isn't, both of them will thank you for stepping up and advocating for them to be allowed the time they need together.

Bottom line – as always, your job is simple: be supportive and encouraging, and help her get the help she needs.

COMPLICATIONS AND INTERVENTIONS
APPENDIX ONE

Like any other major life event, births don't always go the way you plan. Indeed, with birth, it's pretty much guaranteed that something won't happen exactly the way you'd hoped.

Still, it's not helpful to spend your whole time worrying about the many ways in which things can get complicated – because most of them simply aren't going to happen and because you'll be an anxious, emotional wreck if you convince yourself that they are.

If either you or your partner do end up obsessing about a particular outcome, then you should talk it over between yourselves, with her doctor, or even with a counselor, before the big day. That can help you put your concerns in perspective – and, if needed, allow you to make sure that there is, indeed, nothing to be concerned about at present.

One thing that might help is to remember that births tend go the most smoothly when the mom is relaxed – and having her or her partner dwelling on worst case scenarios does not facilitate relaxation.

At the same time, though, we don't advocate an ostrich-in-the-sand approach. It helps to be aware of some of the complications that might arise. So we've listed below some of the most common interventions that can occur in the hospital. This is by no means a comprehensive description of the indications or the risk/benefits of each, but it should give you a place to jump off in discussions with your health care providers.

Induction

Induced labor is when uterine contractions are artificially stimulated before labor begins on its own. The most common drug used for this is Pitocin – so you might hear doctors or other parents talking about deciding to use Pitocin during a birth. That means they want to induce labor. Sometimes, if a mother's cervix is not quite ready for Pitocin to be effective, a doctor might recommend "softening" the cervix first using an artificial prostiglandin.

A healthcare provider can recommend induction for various reasons, but it usually boils down to a concern for either the mother or baby's health. Factors that typically lead to a recommendation to induce include:

- Her water has broken but labor has not begun within 12-24 hours
- The pregnancy is 'post-term' (i.e. it's past 42 weeks)
- The mother has pregnancy-related high blood pressure
- The mother has health problems, such as diabetes, that could affect the baby
- The uterus has signs of infection
- The baby is growing too slowly
- The baby is growing too quickly (due to underlying blood sugar issues, for example)

In theory, doing something that speeds labor along and allows you to meet your baby all the sooner may sound great. And, of course, if it's recommended to you, it's likely the best choice. But inducing labor before a woman begins it of her own accord does increase the risk that the following further interventions will be needed:

- A vacuum- or forceps-assisted vaginal birth
- Administration of an epidural or other drug for pain relief
- Cesarean surgery
- Admission of the baby to an intensive care unit
- Longer hospital stays

Meconium

This is a sticky black substance that is the baby's first bowel movement. It is not uncommon for a baby to poop out its meconium while still in utero, and while that can be an indication of fetal distress, it's more likely just the result of the baby needing to go.

Passing meconium while still inside is not usually a problem for infants, but after they are born and need to breathe, it is not something you want them to inhale. In particular, it can impact the infant's respiration -- so if there is meconium present in a woman's amniotic fluid, the doctor or midwife will typically cut the cord and take the baby to warming table to suction out the nose and mouth instead of putting the baby directly on the mom's belly.

The presence of meconium might also bring more personnel in the room in order to carry out the suctioning – that's simply standard procedure, though, and doesn't mean there is any major emergency.

C-section

Most women hope to have a vaginal birth and avoid surgery, but Cesareans today account for over 30% of births, which makes such a delivery a distinct possibility for all.

Couples often worry about an emergency arising that will cause a panicked and hurried trip to the operating room. While that does happen, it's very rare. The much more typical scenario that results in a Caesarean birth is one that builds over time.

The fundamental issue could be a rising maternal fever, a stop in cervical dilation, a baby that seems to be dealing less and less well with the labor. Situations like these typically give you time to ask questions and get clear why a Caesarian is being considered – allowing you to be comfortable with the notion that this is the best way to bring your baby into the world.

In almost all cases, the birth partner can go with the mom into the operating room. Before she has a cesarean delivery, a nurse will prepare the mom for the operation. An intravenous line gets placed in a vein in her arm or hand to deliver fluids and medications during the surgery. Her belly gets washed and her pubic hair may be clipped or trimmed. She'll also get medication to prevent infection.

A catheter (tube) is placed in her urethra to drain her bladder. Having an empty bladder decreases the chance of injuring it during surgery.

A regional pain block, such as an epidural, is the most commonly used anesthetic here, which means the mom will be awake for the whole thing. Although she won't feel any pain, she's still likely to feel tugs and pulling sensations.

Any surgery carries risks, of course. Among the possible complications from a Cesarean birth are:

- Infection
- Loss of blood
- Blood clots in the legs, pelvic organs, or lungs
- Injury to the bowel or bladder
- A reaction to a medication or to the anesthesia used

You can expect the entire procedure to take about an hour. The actual birth of the baby happens pretty fast, though – the majority of the time is taken up after the birth with the suturing of mom.

Mothers are not usually able to hold their babies immediately after a Cesarean birth due to the constraints of the procedure, but they do get to see them after the babies have been dried, assessed and wrapped up to stay warm. Babies usually then go with the dad or birth partner to the nursery for observation and are reunited with mom in recovery after the surgery is over.

Interventions for an assisted delivery

Sometimes a mother needs some extra help pushing the baby out during a vaginal delivery, usually because she's either too exhausted to push or because her medications are making muscle control difficult.

There are a variety of ways that can happen. Here are the three most common methods:

Vacuum extractor

This is a flexible plastic cup with a handle attached to its underside that gets placed on the baby's head while in the birth canal. The cup is connected by a tube to a vacuum that creates enough suction power to hold the cup onto the head. As the laboring mom experiences a contraction, the doctor pulls gently on the handle – hopefully adding sufficient extra force to help move the baby down and out of the birth canal.

Serious complications from this procedure are pretty rare. Using a vacuum can leave a raised bruise on the baby's head, but it typically goes away within a few weeks or so. That bruise has been found to increase the child's risk of developing jaundice, however, so that needs to be watched for.

Forceps

These are tongs shaped rather like a pair of serving spoons that are slid into the birth canal in order to grasp the baby's head. As with the vacuum, the doctor or midwife gently squeezes the forceps to grip the baby's head and pulls as the mother contracts.

Forceps can also cause bruising, which typically clears up in a few days. There is a risk of facial nerve injury, although that also usually clears up quickly. More serious problems are also possible from the use of forceps, but they are rare and more of a concern for the mother than the child. A forceps delivery can increase the risk of tearing to the mother's cervix, vagina, perineum, and anal sphincter.

Episiotomy

This is a surgical cut made in the perineum, which is the area between the vagina and the anus. It's done immediately prior to delivery in order to give the infant more space to come through.

Episiotomies used to be routine – they were thought to help speed delivery and prevent muscle tears. In addition, a "clean" incision was thought to heal faster than a spontaneous tear and was believed to helped prevent later complications, such as incontinence.

More recent studies find no good evidence that episiotomies are especially protective and suggest that they might even lead to longer healing times, infections and bigger tears. For this reason, the American College of Obstetricians and Gynecologists as well as many other experts now recommend the procedure only be used in cases where the baby truly needs to be born more quickly.

A SAMPLE BIRTH PLAN
APPENDIX TWO

A few words on crafting a birth plan:

Shorter is better. No one will read a manifesto, and then your wishes will be lost.

Make it easy on the eyes for maximum impact. Bullet Points are your friends. And remember: you'll catch more flies with honey than vinegar (the hospital staff are flies and your words are the honey… well, you get the idea). A pleasant tone goes a long way and if you start out strident, you have nowhere to go.

SAMPLE BIRTH PLAN – JANE AND JOHN SMITH

(Intro: tell them a little about you)

Our baby is a boy and at this point we are planning on naming him Lima Bean. Jane is very queasy about needles and we would like to have as few as possible. We are excited to be delivering here and hope to have a healthy happy birth. Thank you for your care.

DURING LABOR AND DELIVERY:

We are hoping for an un-medicated, vaginal delivery and to that end Jane would like to:

- Have as much freedom to move around and choose comfortable positions throughout her labor.
- Have intermittent monitoring if all seems well with the baby.
- Avoid an I.V. (and heparin lock) unless something about the birth would make this unsafe.
- Not be offered pain medication. Jane will let you know if she needs it.
- Be allowed to choose positions for pushing that feel most comfortable and to be guided in Jane's pushing to help minimize tearing.

Cesarean Delivery

If a cesarean becomes necessary it is very important to Jane that John be present with her in the O.R. and that he accompany the baby to the nursery.

POSTPARTUM:

Umbilical Cord

John doesn't care to cut the cord; please wait until it has stopped pulsing to cut it

Medical procedures on baby

- We would like to delay eye medication and vitamin K shot until after initial bonding is established.

- Likewise, we would like to delay blood test (PKU)--if possible, until the first doctor's visit.

- If baby must be taken from room, and/or if medical procedures must be performed on the baby, either John or Jane would like to accompany the baby at all times.

Rooming-in

We plan to room-in with the baby 24 hours a day and have requested a private room.

A HOSPITAL PACK LIST
APPENDIX THREE

This is by no means a comprehensive list, but it does cover the basics. These are all items that you're likely to want with you when you are in the hospital. In the case of the car seat, most facilities won't let you drive the baby home without one:

Personal care:
- Toiletries for both of you: toothbrush, glasses and contact care, hairbrush, mints, hair ties, lip balm
- Shower supplies

Food and drink:
- Snacks for partner and for mom (cheese sticks, crackers, energy bars, fruit).
- Anything you'd like to drink besides water and juice (e.g. Gatorade, Recharge, broth mixes)

Clothing:
- For her: warm socks, robe, underwear, clothes to go home in (remember, she will still have a tummy).
- Shower shoes/flip-flops
- Baby: hat, outfit, blanket and diaper/s
- Partner: Clothes for your hospital stay

Comfort supplies:
- Birth ball
- Lotion
- Massage tools

- Heat pack
- Music player
- Focal Point

Misc.:
- Camera
- Car seat
- Copy of this book (!)
- Cell phones and chargers
- Books and magazines

ENDNOTES

About the authors *(in case you skipped this earlier!)*

Julie Dubrouillet is a certified labor support doula, childbirth and lactation educator and prenatal yoga instructor, as well as a trainer of childbirth educators. She is also the pre-natal Health Education Specialist at the Palo Alto Medical Foundation in Palo Alto, California. A mother of two children, she's taught thousands of couples how best to approach childbirth and directly supported hundreds of couples through the births of their children.

Simon Firth is a writer specializing in stories about parenting and technology. He's written for Salon, Wondertime, Food and Wine and the Christian Science Monitor among other publications and is a regular technology analyst for the London Evening Standard. He attended the births of his two children, where he lovingly supported his wife thanks to the tips he learned in a class taught by Julie! Julie was also the doula attending his children's births.

Sara Burgess is an illustrator and designer. You can see more of her work at www.whitepaperspress.com.

Send us feedback

Again, this is a living document. We want it to keep getting better and better. So let us know what you think could make it even more helpful. Write to us at deliverbook@yahoo.com and tell us what else you'd like us to cover or how else we could be a help.

Other resources

If you're interested in finding other reputable books and websites that explore pregnancy, childbirth and labor assistance, check the recommendations on our web page, www.deliverbook.com.

You'll also find links there to music that you might consider adding to your labor playlists, and our birth-related blog.

Made in the USA
San Bernardino, CA
06 December 2018